Leaky Gut Diet

The FODMAP Diet Made Easy - Simple solutions for IBS and Bowel Disorders

© **Copyright 2018 - All rights reserved.**

The contents of this book may not be reproduced, duplicated or transmitted without direct written permission from the author.

Under no circumstances will any legal responsibility or blame be held against the publisher for any reparation, damages, or monetary loss due to the information herein, either directly or indirectly.

Legal Notice:

You cannot amend, distribute, sell, use, quote or paraphrase any part or the content within this book without the consent of the author.

Disclaimer Notice:

Please note the information contained within this document is for educational and entertainment purposes only. No warranties of any kind are expressed or implied. Readers acknowledge that the author is not engaging in the rendering of legal, financial, medical or professional advice. Please consult a licensed professional before attempting any techniques outlined in this book.

By reading this document, the reader agrees that under no circumstances are is the author responsible for any losses, direct or indirect, which are incurred as a result of the use of information contained within this document, including, but not limited to, —errors, omissions, or inaccuracies.

Table of Contents
Introduction
Chapter One: An Introduction to Irritable Bowel Syndrome and the FODMAP diet
   Irritable Bowel Syndrome (IBS) – What is it?
     Symptoms of IBS
   Low FODMAP diet – What is it?
Chapter Two: Symptoms of FODAMP Explained
Chapter Three – Diagnosis of the Irritable Bowel Syndrome
Chapter Four – Foods to Eat on a Low FODMAP Diet
   Foods to avoid or reduce completely
     Veggies and legumes –
     Fruits – they can contain high amounts of fructose
     Meats, meat substitutes, poultry
     Grains, cereals, biscuits, nuts, pasta, and cakes
     Bread
     Dips, condiments, sweeteners, sweets, and spreads
     Sweeteners
     Prebiotic foods
     Protein powders and drinks
     Teas
     Fennel tea
     Dairy based products
     Milk
     Cooking ingredients –
   Foods to consume
     Vegetables and legumes
     Fruits
     Meats, meat substitutes, and poultry
     Seafood and fish
     Grains, cereals, biscuits, nuts, pasta, and cakes
     Bread
     Rice
     Seeds –
     Condiments, sweets, dips, spreads, and sweeteners
     Protein powders and drinks

    Dairy products and eggs
    Herbs, spices, and cooking ingredients
Chapter Five: Common Mistakes Made by People When on a Low FODMAP Diet
    Eating a lot at once
    Consuming processed food products
    Holding on for prolonged periods of time
    Having unrealistic expectations
    Making all changes in one go
    An Inadequate Intake of Fiber
    When you over-limit your diet
Chapter Six: Natural Methods to Reduce Irritable Bowel Syndrome Symptoms
    Drinking ample amounts of water
    Peppermint oil based supplements
    Reduce your levels of stress
    Try not to be sedentary
    Consuming herbal teas to alleviate Irritable Bowel Syndrome symptoms
Chapter Seven: Meal Plan Ideas
    Sunday
    Monday
    Tuesday
    Wednesday
    Thursday
    Friday
    Saturday
Chapter Eight: The Low FODMAP Diet and Weight Loss
    Practice being lenient towards yourself
    Maintain a food diary for several days or a week
    Adding more fruits and veggies to your snacks and over all meals
    Focus on the can haves and not the can't haves of your diet
    Planning ahead

Chapter Nine: Tips for Eating out when on the Low FODMAP Diet
    It's the low FODMAP, not a no FODMAP diet!
    Ensure checking the menu beforehand
    Informing a restaurant of your intolerances
    Pick the dishes that are the safe and try making adaptations if required
    Be watchful of the serving size, sugar, and fat
    You've upset your stomach – what now?

Chapter Ten: Reincorporating FODMAPs Back into Your Dietary Habits

Chapter Eleven: Breakfast Recipes
    Baked Oatmeal Cups
    Breakfast Cereal Bars
    Breakfast Potatoes
    Blueberry Kiwi Minty Groovy Smoothie
    Pineapple Ginger Kale Smoothie
    Potato Scones

Chapter Twelve: Snack Recipes
    Carrot and Parsnip Chips
    Bacon Wrapped Pineapple
    Roasted Chickpeas
    Cucumber and Dill-infused Cottage Cheese Appetizer

Chapter Thirteen: Lunch Recipes
    Potato Salad with Anchovy and Quail's Eggs
    Low FODMAP Chicken Noodle Soup
    Egg Wraps
    Poached Egg Sandwich with Smoked Salmon
    Buckwheat Pancakes

Chapter Fourteen: Dinner Recipes
    Sweet and Sour Chicken
    Baked Lemon Pepper Chicken & Rice
    Beef Skillet Supper
    Sardine Spaghetti with Tomato- Caper Sauce
    Spiced Quinoa with Almonds and Feta
    Vegan Coconut Green Curry

    Spicy Potato Pie
Chapter Fifteen: Dessert Recipes
    Banana Ice Cream
    Chocolate Peanut Butter Chia Pudding
    Frosted Biscotti
    Chocolate Coconut Cookies
Chapter Sixteen: Dip Recipes
    Arugula Feta Dip
    FODMAP Friendly Hummus
    Berry Chia Jam
Conclusion
Resources

Introduction

I want to thank you for choosing this book, *'Leaky Gut Diet - The FODMAP Diet Made Easy - Simple solutions for IBS and Bowel Disorders'* and I assure you that you have made the right choice in choosing this book.

This book is perfect for people suffering from bloating, severe diarrhea and constipation in their everyday lives. If you are unable to understand these problems completely or figure out how to go about the low FODMAP diet that you have heard about as the solution to Irritable Bowel Syndrome related symptoms, then you have come to the right place!

This book has been crafted to better your understanding of the low FODMAP diet, all the symptoms involved, how to go about meals, and various other helpful information has been covered – along with a section of recipes to get you started!

I wish you luck on your low FODMAP journey.

Thank you!

Chapter One: An Introduction to Irritable Bowel Syndrome and the FODMAP diet

Irritable Bowel Syndrome (IBS) – What is it?

Irritable Bowel Syndrome is a type of medical condition where the sufferer experiences constipation, abdominal pain, diarrhea, bloating and irregular bowel movements. So far, the exact reason or cause of this medical condition has not been found. There are specific factors that could lead to having an irritable bowel – factors like consuming vast amounts of junk foods or neglecting your water intake which can lead to a lack of hydration. Some other causes are excessive amounts of stress, family history, etc.

As Irritable Bowel Syndrome symptoms start getting extreme, the patients pass blood via their stools. If you have been suffering or someone you know has been experiencing such extreme levels of IBS symptoms – hurry! You need to rush to a doctor immediately and begin the appropriate line or method of treatment. If this condition is left untreated for long periods of time, it will start disrupting the quality of the life you lead. It could potentially become something that prevents you from living a normal and healthy life.

Symptoms of IBS

People who have Irritable Bowel Syndrome could experience symptoms such as –

- Diarrhea – most often this is described as episodes of diarrhea that are rather violent.
- Constipation.
- Constipation that keeps alternating with diarrhea.
- Immense amounts of bloating or even gas problems.
- A lot of belly cramps and pains, mostly in the belly's lower half region. These cramps and pains tend to get worse after an intake of meals, but are relieved or improved following a bowel movement.
- A tummy that tends to stick out a lot.
- Symptoms can be made worse with excessive stress. Patients of IBS are advised to avoid worrying too much as it can only worsen their condition.
- Stools that are looser or harder than normal (flat ribbon or pellet stools)
- There are also individuals who experience sexual problems or urinary symptoms.

There exist four kinds of the Irritable Bowel Syndrome.

- Irritable Bowel Syndrome with Constipation: IBS-C
- Irritable Bowel Syndrome with Diarrhea: IBS-D
- There are people who experience a pattern that keeps alternating between diarrhea and constipation. This mixed condition of the Irritable Bowel Syndrome is called IBS-M.
- Individuals who experience IBS symptoms that fit into none of the categories listed above are called unsubtyped Irritable Bowel Syndrome, or IBS-U.

Low FODMAP diet – What is it?

FODMAP – Fermentable Oligosaccharides, Disaccharides, Monosaccharides and Polyols

All of these terms that FODMAP consists of have been named after specific and complex molecules. These molecules are found in foods that some individuals might find tough to absorb. This very lack of absorption that occurs in the intestinal tract might let harmful bacteria gather in the stomach. That will eventually lead to medical conditions like irritable bowel, or the IBS that you were briefed about in the preceding section.

The low FODMAP diet is the kind of diet that helps reduce many types of bowel related problems people might be facing. Along with that, it helps with issues like Crohn's disease or other similar tummy related issues.

Chapter Two: Symptoms of FODAMP Explained

<u>Meals become synonymous with bloating</u>

FODMAP ingredients like fructose usually tend to be absorbed easily via the small intestine. However, for some people, this easy feat is an extremely difficult experience. What happens is that when the fructose goes into the large intestine, it pretty much ends up being treated like a foreign entity. That often results in more bacteria being created down into the gut. Not only that, but this problem could aggravate further and turn into diarrhea, constipation, and also bloating that is constant.

There are people who experience extreme amounts of pain in the gut area, which is directly caused by the formation of excessive amounts of gas. This kind of intolerance generally becomes the reason multiple problems in the body end up being created. Problems apply especially in the form of restlessness, lack of sleep and even fatigue. People who suffer from this type of intolerance generally cringe even at the thought of food or the idea of consuming it, since the effects they experience after consuming food become immensely tough to tolerate.

Foods that are generally thought to be healthy only end up worsening the existing symptoms

A lot of people, and even experts tend to believe that foods that are healthy refers to every kind of fruit, vegetable, whole grain and legume. While out of all these ingredients some are definitely helpful, a lot of them could emerge as very problematic and harmful. That is especially for individuals who suffer from problems like an irritable bowel. The reason behind this is that all of these foods have a pretty high level of fructose in them. That makes it tough for the foods to be digested.

While there do exist foods that have a much lower content of fructose, most of the others contain marginally high quantities of it. This is why it is so essential to be aware of which kinds of foods are included in the low FODMAP category. It is always advisable to look up whether or not an ingredient is a part of the low FODMAP category before you even think of buying - or worse – consuming it. If you have been experiencing any of the symptoms that have been explained in this section of the book then be extra careful.

It is important to note that whole grains, which are especially considered as healthy, in fact, contain high amounts of fructans. This is why they need to be avoided in order to diminish the symptoms.

Lactose intolerance is not a part of it, but it is recommended to avoid not consume it

Anyone who is suffering from FODMAP issues may not be intolerant towards lactose. Some, in fact, may not have any problems related to dairy based products at all. But it is rather helpful to remove dairy based products from your everyday diet. They could just as well add to irritable bowel problems you could be facing, to an extent. The thing is that dairy products could be absolutely no problem to you. You might assume continuing to consume these products will not cause any harm to your health. But it is highly possible that you might end up suffering from dairy based intolerance sometime soon or in the future. It's better if you stay safe than to regret it later.

Being unable to identify the reason or cause

There are a lot of people who spend years of their lives struggling with bloating problems without realizing what exactly has been causing it. Generally, people don't bother or care enough to look into the problem. That is of course unless other or different symptoms start manifesting or when the bloating reaches a stage that is unbearable. People even develop the habit of searching for the symptoms on the Internet for such problems and then try to diagnose the problem by themselves.

Although the advent of technology has done a lot of good things for us, it has also, in a lot of ways, misled people in regards to many things. It is important to understand things like info we gather from the Internet. This is only able to serve us to a specific extent. There is no way it can surpass years and decades of experience that a doctor can offer you. So the next time a symptom manifests make sure your first priority is to get checked by a doctor without any delay. There should be no reason for you to compromise on your health or the quality of life you are leading.

In the case of consulting a doctor not being of any help

Not every doctor is going to be able to identify symptoms that are linked with Irritable Bowel Syndrome. Although it is not something that occurs often, it is possible that the doctor you consult might not be able to diagnose the reason behind your symptoms. So what should you do in such a scenario? All you can do is learn as much as possible about the symptoms you are experiencing by observing things like what soothes the symptoms or what worsens them.

If your doctor has recommended adding more fiber to your diet, do not begin eating all kinds of veggies and fruits. It would be dangerous to have zero consideration towards following or even checking the low FODMAP chart. In fact, this could exacerbate the issue instead of solving it, simply as a result of not specifically choosing the low FODMAP fruits and veggies.

The majority of doctors do not recommend nutritional training, although it will play an important role when it comes to your recovery. Also, apart from consulting a doctor, you could also seek help from certified nutritionists in order to reduce the IBS symptoms.

Rushing to the washroom far too frequently

A lot of the people who are suffering from an irritable bowel tend to experience extreme cases of diarrhea or constipation. Constipation happens as a result of a lack of intake of either fiber or water in the body. When the body is experiencing a lack of hydration, it makes the bowel content dry up. This causes them to move at a slower pace. Extreme cases of constipation related problems could make it tough for someone to pass stools. That could eventually result in fistula, hemorrhoids and anal fissures.

Diarrhea is a result of excessive amounts of liquid entering your bowels. This ends up making the food to move at an accelerated pace through the bowels. That does not allow enough time to let the regular process of the colon drying out. If diarrheal infection stays around for longer periods of time, then this could lead to other problems like an inflammation of the colon. That will only pave the road to more bacteria gathering in your bowel.

If you are constantly feeling the urge to empty your bowel, then it is a major sign something is not quite right with your bowel. Just this one symptom is enough for someone to realize that it is of utmost importance to consult a doctor as soon as possible.

Your digestion problems have started hampering your life

When you are a sufferer of an irritable bowel, it will seem as if the reins of your life have been handed to this problem. For example, the thought of attending a social gathering could seem like a mountainous task to achieve as it involves having to eat heavy foods. It might even be a matter of concern since it would mean you might need to use the washroom pretty often while at such gatherings. It could get a bit embarrassing, either for you or pretty much everyone including you.

When your gut seems to be malfunctioning, you will always tend to struggle with leaning towards your favorite foods. Having an irritable bowel might also bother your regular sleeping patterns, and leave you feeling fatigued pretty much all of the time. Maybe you will also experience sleepiness throughout the day. If you have been experiencing any of the symptoms mentioned in this chapter, rush to consult a doctor or a general physician who knows your history.

Chapter Three – Diagnosis of the Irritable Bowel Syndrome

Irritable bowel is a condition that is kind of difficult to identify. The majority of people in the United States tend to suffer from digestive disorders on a pretty frequent basis. That is a result of unhealthy food related habits. There is no specific test that can possible diagnose irritable bowel syndrome. In fact, it is only possible to detect via incessant symptoms in regards to problems associated with the digestive system.

When you consult a general physician, you find that doctors will ask their patients to observe what could possibly be triggering the symptoms. One vital rule of thumb is gathering all information related to any irritable bowel problems present in your family history. The doctor will also ask you about how often you experience the symptoms or how often they manifest. Along with that – how long does it take for the symptoms to go away? Only then will they be able to form a proper analysis about what's going on with you and your bowel.

It is required of you to make sure you are completely cooperating with your doctor to help him figure out a diagnosis that is accurate. One of your best bets would be to jot down all of your symptoms to form a list. Be sure to note down what you are experiencing, how frequently, how long it lasts, and what makes the symptoms go away. It will just take a piece of paper and a pen or pencil and it will save you and your doctor a lot of time. Not only that but it will also ensure you do not leave out any vital pieces of information that need to be conveyed to the doctor.

Here are some of the questions most commonly asked by doctors in regard to irritable bowel problems:

- Do you feel a reduction in abdominal pains after emptying your bowel?
- How often do you feel the urge to defecate or urinate?
- How stressful would you say your everyday life is? Are the symptoms aggravated by excessive stress?
- Do your stools seem to appear different in any manner on the days you experience the symptoms?
- How painful would you say it gets while passing stools?
- Does consuming heavy meals make your tummy feel gassy or get bloated?
- Do you drink enough water? How much water do you drink on a daily basis?

- How often do you work out or engage in any exercise or sporty activity?
- Do you experience any dip in your levels of energy when the symptoms manifest?
- Have you taken any kind of medication for the irritable bowel problems you are facing?
- Has your sleep been affected by these symptoms?
- How irritable or anxious do you tend to feel throughout the course of a day?

Once you have answered all the questions posed by the doctor to the best of your ability, you will be advised on the required line of treatment. That could include – changing your everyday diet, taking antibiotics or regular physically engaging activities. Maybe even a change in the lifestyle you are leading will be necessary. If you do intend to cure the bowel problems you are facing, it is essential you stay on track with the doctor's suggested line of treatment. If you follow the treatment even if for just one month, you will start noticing positive differences with your condition very soon.

Chapter Four – Foods to Eat on a Low FODMAP Diet

What FODMAP consists of is sugars that are not digestible easily, which could wreck your bowel or wreak havoc on it.

F – Fermentable

Fermentable refers to the breaking down process of carbohydrates by the gut bacteria. When they are not digested, they produce gases like hydrogen, carbon dioxide or methane.

O – Olgio saccharides

Fructans or fructo-oligosacharides or Galacto-oligosaccharides

D – Disaccharides

Lactose

M – Monosaccharide

Fructose

Polyols

What these include is sugar Polyols like sorbitol and Mannitol.

Here is a list of ingredients that are required for consumption when on a low FODMAP diet along with the foods you should avoid. It would be an impossible task to list down nearly all foods. So, mentioned below is a list of ingredients to better your understanding and guide you into choosing better food for your condition.

Foods to avoid or reduce completely

Veggies and legumes –

- Artichoke
- Baked beans
- Ripe bananas
- Asparagus
- Fresh beetroot
- Broad beans
- Cauliflower
- Cassava
- Choko
- Celery – stalk that is greater than 5cm
- Butter beans
- Black eyed peas –
- Black beans
- Fermented cabbage, like sauerkraut
- Falafel
- Haricot beans
- Lima beans
- Kidney beans
- Mange tout
- Mung beans
- Leek bulb
- Mixed vegetables
- Peas, sugar snap
- Mushrooms
- Red kidney beans
- Soy beans / soya beans
- Spring onions / scallions (white part / bulb)

- Pickled vegetables
- Savoy cabbage
- Taro
- Shallots
- Split peas

Fruits – they can contain high amounts of fructose

- Apricots
- Apples
- Blackberries
- Avocado
- Blackcurrants
- Cherries
- Currants
- Dates
- Grapefruit
- Litchi
- Guava
- Figs
- Feijao
- Boysenberry
- Custards apple
- Goji berries
- Nectarines
- Mango
- Pears
- Paw paw, dried
- Persimmon
- Plums
- Pineapple, dried

- Pomegranate
- Sea buckthorns
- Watermelon
- Tinned fruit in pear or apple juice
- Tamarillo
- Sultanas
- Raisins
- Peaches

Meats, meat substitutes, poultry

- Sausages
- Chorizo

Grains, cereals, biscuits, nuts, pasta, and cakes

- Wheat based products –
- Wheat, bread – more than a slice
- Cookies, including choco chip cookies
- Breadcrumbs
- Wheat based cereal bar
- Crumpets
- Croissants
- Egg noodles
- Cakes
- Pastries
- Muffins
- Udon noodles – more than ½ cup
- Wheat cereal
- Wheat bran
- Wheat flour

- Wheat rolls
- Wheat noodles
- Wheat germ
- Almond meal
- Barley, as well as barley flour
- Amaranth flour
- Almond meal
- Couscous
- Freekeh
- Muesli bar
- Rye
- Pistachios
- Semolina
- Rye crisp bread
- Gnocchi
- Muesli cereal
- Einkorn flour
- Cashews
- Bran cereals

Bread

- Multigrain bread
- Roti
- Granary bread
- Naan
- Pumpernickel bread
- Sourdough with kamut
- Oatmeal bread

Dips, condiments, sweeteners, sweets, and spreads

- Caviar dip
- Agave
- High fructose corn syrup (HFCS)
- Honey
- Hummus
- Pesto sauce
- Quince paste
- Vegetable pickle / relish
- Jam, strawberry – if it has HFCS
- Jam, mixed berries
- Gravy – if the ingredients contain onion
- Fruit bar
- Stock cubes
- Tahini paste
- Sugar free sweets that contain Polyols – normally ending with Isomalt or –ol

Sweeteners

- Isomalt
- Inulin
- Maltitol
- Xylitol
- Sorbitol
- Mannitol

Prebiotic foods

These items could be hiding in snack bars, yogurts, etc. –
- Inulin

- Oligofructose
- FOS – fructo-oligosacharides

Protein powders and drinks

- Coconut water
- Cordial – raspberry and apple - 50 to 200 percent of real juice
- Kombucha
- Rum
- Chocolate flavored drink – malted
- Fruit juice in high quantities
- Sports drinks
- Wine – more than a glass
- Sodas that contain High Fructose Corn Syrup
- Fruit juices made of pear, apple, and mango
- Orange juice – exceeding 100ml in quantity
- Whey protein – lactose free or hydrolyzed
- Cordial – orange – 25 to 50 percent of real juice
- Whey protein, lactose free or concentrate
- Beer – if consuming more than one bottle
- Soy milk produced with soy beans
- Herbal and fruit teas with added apple

Teas

- Chai that has a strong flavor
- Black tea with soy milk added to it

Fennel tea

- Dandelion tea that has a strong flavor
- Herbal tea that has a strong flavor

- Chamomile tea that has a strong flavor
- Oolong tea

Dairy based products

- Kefir
- Cream
- Gelato
- Custard
- Cream cheese
- Ricotta cheese
- Halloumi
- Ice cream
- Yogurt
- Sour cream

Milk

- Goat milk
- Cow milk
- Sheep's milk
- Evaporated milk

Cooking ingredients –

- Carob powder

Foods to consume

Vegetables and legumes

- Alfalfa
- Bean sprouts
- Bok choy

- Bamboo shoots
- Bitter gourd
- Broccoli, whole – one cup
- Broccoli, only stalks – one cup
- Broccoli, only heads – one cup
- Butternut squash – a quarter of a cup
- Brussels sprouts – one serving of 2 sprouts
- Cabbage, red and common – up to one cup
- Carrots
- Callaloo
- Celery – less than or not more than 5cm of a stalk
- Celeriac
- Cho cho
- Choy sum
- Courgette
- Corn or sweet corn – but only if tolerable and only in less amounts – half of a cob
- Collard greens
- Chives
- Chili – only if it is tolerable
- Chick peas – a quarter of a cup
- Chicory leaves
- Eggplant or aubergine
- Green pepper / green capsicum / green bell pepper
- Ginger
- Green beans
- Kale
- Leek leaves
- Okra
- Marrow
- Parsnip
- Olives

- Snow peas – five pods
- Pickled onions, large
- Pickled gherkins
- Canned pumpkin – a quarter of a cup or 2.2 ounces
- Potato
- Radish
- Pumpkin
- Seaweed or nori
- Squash
- Baby spinach
- Chard or silverbeet
- Spring onions or scallions (only the green part)
- Red bell peppers or red capsicum or red peppers
- Spaghetti squash
- Swede
- Swiss chard
- Sun-dried tomatoes – up to 4 pieces only
- Sweet potato – not more than half cup
- Turnip
- Tomato – cherry, common, roma, and canned
- Yam
- Zucchini
- Water chestnuts
- Lettuce – iceberg lettuce, butter lettuce, radicchio lettuce, rocket lettuce, red coral lettuce

Fruits

- Ackee
- Bilberries
- Unripe bananas

- Breadfruit
- Blueberries
- Cantaloupe
- Carambola
- Clementine
- Cranberry – one tablespoon
- Dragon fruit
- Grapes
- Lingonberries
- Ripe guava
- Kiwifruit
- Gaila melons and honeydew
- Lime as well as lime juice
- Lemon as well as lemon juice
- Orange
- Mandarin
- Passion fruit
- Pineapple
- Papaya
- Plantain, peeled
- Rhubarb
- Raspberry
- Tamarind
- Strawberry
- Paw paw
- Tangelo

Meats, meat substitutes, and poultry

- Chicken
- Beef

- Lamb
- Prosciutto
- Quorn, mince
- Processed meat – but check the ingredients
- Turkey
- Cold cuts or deli meats or cold meats like turkey breast and ham

Seafood and fish

- Haddock
- Cod
- Salmon
- Plaice
- Trout
- Tuna
- Canned tuna

Seafood (but make sure nothing else is included) –

- Lobster
- Crab
- Oysters
- Shrimp
- Prawns
- Mussels

Grains, cereals, biscuits, nuts, pasta, and cakes

- Gluten free breads
- Wheat free breads

Bread

- Oat bread
- Corn bread
- Rice bread
- Potato flour bread
- Spelt sourdough bread

- Gluten free or wheat free pasta
- Wheat bread – one slice
- Shortbread cookie – only one
- Savory cookie
- Almonds – a maximum of 15
- Brazil nuts
- Buckwheat
- Buckwheat noodles
- Buckwheat flour
- Whole grain rice or brown rice
- Plain chips or plain potato crisps
- Chestnuts
- Cornflakes – half cup
- Crisp bread
- Maize or corn flour
- Corn tortillas – three tortillas
- Coconut – milk and cream but fresh
- Bulgur / bourghal – a quarter cup, but cooked
- Plain crackers

- Millet
- Macadamia nuts
- Mixed nuts
- Oatcakes
- Oatmeal – half cup
- Oats
- Peanuts
- Hazelnuts – a maximum of 5
- Pecans – a maximum of 15
- Polenta
- Pine nuts – a maximum of 15
- Popcorn
- Potato flour
- Quinoa
- Pretzels
- Oat based cereals and porridge
- Wheat pasta – up to half cup and cooked

Rice

- Brown rice
- Basmati rice
- White rice
- Rice noodles
- Rice cakes
- Rice bran
- Rice crackers
- Rice flour
- Rice flakes
- Rice Crispies

Seeds –

- Egusi seeds

- Chia seeds
- Poppy seeds
- Sesame seeds
- Pumpkin seeds
- Sunflower seeds
- Maize, starch, tapioca, and potato
- Tortilla chips or corn chips
- Sorghum
- Walnuts

Condiments, sweets, dips, spreads, and sweeteners

- Acesulfame K
- Aspartame
- Barbecue sauce – read label carefully for the ingredients
- Salted capers
- Capers in vinegar
- Chutney – one tablespoon
- Milk chocolate – three squares
- Dark chocolate
- White chocolate – three squares
- Glucose
- Golden syrup
- Maple syrup
- Mustard
- Miso paste
- Ketchup – one sachet
- Fish sauce
- Marmite

- Marmalade
- Mayonnaise – make sure it contains neither onion nor garlic
- Jelly or jam, strawberry
- Pesto sauce – less than a tablespoon
- Oyster sauce
- Wasabi
- Tomato sauce – two sachets
- Vegemite
- Tamarind paste
- Stevia
- Soy sauce
- Peanut butter
- Saccharine
- Rice malt syrup
- Worcestershire sauce – contains both onion and garlic but in extremely low amounts which makes it low FODMAP
- Balsamic vinegar – two tablespoons
- Apple cider vinegar – two tablespoons
- Rice wine vinegar
- Sucralose
- Shrimp paste
- Sweet and sour sauce
- Sugar – also known as sucrose

Protein powders and drinks

Alcohol – to the gut it is an irritant and only limited intake is recommended
- Beer – limit it to one drink

- Gin
- Wine – limit to one drink
- Whiskey
- Clear spirits like vodka

Coffee
- Espresso coffee, decaffeinated or regular – black
- Espresso coffee, decaffeinated or regular, with lactose free milk up to 250ml
- Instant coffee, decaffeinated or regular, with lactose free milk up to 250ml
- Instant coffee, decaffeinated or regular, black

- Fruit juice up to 125ml and only consume safe fruit
- Lemonade – in low amounts
- Drinking chocolate powder
- Kvass

Protein powders –
- Pea protein – 20g
- Egg protein
- Rice protein
- Whey protein
- Sacha inchi protein

- Soy milk produced from soy protein

Tea

- Black tea, but weak
- Herbal and fruit tea, weak and without adding any apple
- Peppermint tea
- Green tea
- White tea

Soft drinks or sodas that contain no high fructose corn syrup or HFCS – like cola, lemonade, etc. but make sure you consume them in limited quantities since these can be unhealthy generally and could also result in gut irritation.

Sodas or soft drinks like diet cokes, but ensure you consume them in low quantities since Acesulfame k and aspartame can be irritants.

Water

Dairy products and eggs

- Dairy free chocolate pudding
- Margarine
- Eggs

Cheese –

- Camembert
- Brie
- Feta
- Ricotta – two tablespoons
- Parmesan
- Mozzarella
- Cheddar
- Swiss cheese
- Chevre or goat

- Soy protein (but do avoid soy beans)
- Tempeh
- Whipped cream
- Goat yogurt
- Lactose free yogurt

- Greek yogurt – in small quantities
- Sorbet

Milk
- Hemp milk
- Almond milk
- Rice milk – maximum limit of 200ml for each sitting
- Oat milk – 30ml which should be enough for cereal
- Almond milk

Herbs, spices, and cooking ingredients

Herbs –
- Cilantro
- Basil
- Curry leaves
- Coriander
- Lemongrass
- Gotukala
- Mint
- Pandan
- Oregano
- Parsley
- Rosemary
- Rampa
- Thyme
- Tarragon
- Sage
- Bay leaves
- Fenugreek

Spices

- Cardamom
- Allspice
- Cloves
- Black pepper
- Five spice
- Cinnamon
- Chili powder (do check the ingredient one, sometimes they contain garlic)
- Saffron
- Turmeric
- Star anise
- Mustard seeds
- Nutmeg
- Fennel seeds
- Cumin
- Paprika

Oils

- Coconut oil
- Peanut oil
- Olive oil
- Rice bran oil
- Canola oil
- Avocado oil
- Coconut oil
- Soybean oil
- Sesame oil
- Vegetable oil
- Sunflower oil
- Onion infused oil

- Garlic infused oil
- Baking soda
- Baking powder
- Cocoa powder
- Gelatin
- Icing sugar
- Ghee
- Lard
- Cream – half cup
- Salt
- Asafetida powder – a really good substitute for onion

Chapter Five: Common Mistakes Made by People When on a Low FODMAP Diet

Most of the time, despite putting themselves on a low FODMAP diet, people experience little or no alleviation. The small hope they had of getting their bowel resettled by following the low FODMAP diet will start feeling like an unachievable dream. But what they do not realize is that they might be making fundamental mistakes. These mistakes could be creating hurdles for their recovery. Some common mistakes have been discussed below:

Eating a lot at once

Just because you are on a low FODMAP diet does not mean it is okay to over-eat. It is easy to get ecstatic over how light you feel after consuming foods based on the low FODMAP diet. However, consuming vast amounts of foods at once can put a lot of pressure and strain on your bowel. But that doesn't mean you are supposed to starve yourself or start skipping meals. When it comes to doing it right – the key is to maintain a balance. Make sure you are breaking your meals down and consuming them in smaller amounts in one sitting. This way, it is easier for the gut when it has to break the food down.

It is also very important that you keep yourself hydrated throughout the day and make it a top priority to drink enough water. This is essential for your recovery but you should also be aware of when exactly to drink water. Make sure you consume proper amounts of liquid at least 2 hours prior to eating your meals and one hour after taking your food. Not allowing your intake of liquid to cause any interference with the process of digestion, it lets your gut digest the foods without any strenuous effort. Also, be mindful of the portions of your food when you are eating.

Consuming processed food products

You must stay miles away from any and every kind of processed food product. Make sure you always check the labels when you are buying food products. Look at the ingredients listed to see what is unfamiliar to you. If there is even one ingredient that you have difficulty recognizing, then do not even consider buying that food. Before you start being on a low FODMAP diet you need to make sure of one thing - that your kitchen does not have any such processed foods and is completely free of them. Either throw away or giveaway whatever packaged food items might be present in your kitchen. Never touch such foods ever again. This might sound like an extreme step to you, but you need to do this anyway as packaged foods are poisonous at for your health. Not only that but, in the long run, it could cause a lot of harm as well.

But does that imply you need to discard all the packets of rice flour too? Well, no, that is not required. You do not need to discard products that have just one ingredient like in this case – rice since it only contains rice and no other ingredient. The products you need to remove come with a list of ingredients that is complex. Also, some of those ingredients will even seem entirely unfamiliar when you see
them printed on labels.

Packaged foods like sauces, packaged meat, and ready to make foods all need to be removed right away.

Holding on for prolonged periods of time

There will be scenarios when you are at social gatherings and you are suppressing the urge to rush to the washroom. Think about it - do you really think it's going to be worth it? When you suppress the urge to empty your bowel, you only end up adding a lot more pressure onto your bowel. In fact, in such scenarios, you should never hesitate when it comes to using the washroom as frequently as you want to.

First of all, keep in mind that not everyone is bothered or interested in observing how frequently you visit the washroom. Secondly, even if anyone does, it is up to you to realize how important it is to prioritize your health. Focus on that instead of caring about these trivial things and worrying about what people will think.

The more you hold onto the urge to empty your bowel, the longer it will take you to recover. In fact, holding it in might hamper whatever recovery you might have attained so far. It is entirely up to you to decide whether you want a recovery as soon as possible or to avoid embarrassment and continue to suffer. It's entirely up to you.

Having unrealistic expectations

It is important that the expectations you have of the FODMAP diet are as realistic as possible. Learning as much as you can regarding things like how the body tends to react to FODMAPS could largely help you. It will also empower you in managing your Irritable Bowel Syndrome a lot more effectively. In fact, it will also help in figuring out a lot of things you might be facing because of it.

And it is really important to do that since there are patients who are very grateful for what the FODMAP diet has done for them - especially when they claim that prior to being on the diet, they did not know what being normal or leading a normal life truly felt like.

But it is just as essential to bear in mind that FODMAPs by themselves are not at the root reason for Irritable Bowel Syndrome. Thus, removing them from your diet is not going to cure you condition. However, a lot of people gradually make a return to an altered version of the diet they prefer. You need to recognize that there are some specific kinds of food that you need to learn never to overdo under any circumstances.

Making all changes in one go

If you are making changes to your diet, supplements, and medications all at once, then how will you figure out what did or did not work in your favor? You will most likely end up learning a lot more from your FODMAP removal and reincorporation process, given that you let the rest of your routine habits stay stable for several weeks as you experiment.

You need to work with and cooperate with your other providers of health care in order to negotiate this. Maybe try making a delay in a new prescription that has been proposed for supplements or medication until after the initial weeks of being on the diet. In the case of you being treated with antibiotics for problems like SIBO, Small Intestinal Bacterial Overgrowth, it is usually best done right before you begin a low FODMAP diet.

An Inadequate Intake of Fiber

Your intake of fiber could end up taking a hit when on a low FODMAP diet. That is not ideal as fiber is a very important source of food for the good bacteria residing in your gut. In fact, other than producing gas, these gut bacteria also perform various services that are essential to the health of the human body.

Increasing your fiber intake in a deliberate manner from the foods allowed in the low FODMAP diet works as a solution to this. Try consuming a vast variety of fruit and vegetables that are on the low FODMAP diet. Along with that, also go for legumes and grains that are low FODMAP. Consider nuts and seeds allowed on the low FODMAP diet but make sure you consume them in small servings only.

Fibers that are low FODMAP tend to ferment at a lot slower pace and are not too likely when it comes to disrupting the balance of fluid in the gut.

When you over-limit your diet

Make sure that you are eating a wide variety of foods that are low FODMAP unless there are important reasons for you to not to. For example – lactose is the only component originating from dairy products that should be avoided when doing a low FODMAP diet.

Unless you are allergic to milk products or are vegan, it is okay for you to continue using products that are made with low-lactose milk. You can use lactose free yogurts and cheeses that have been aged, when following a low FODMAP diet.

Also, similarly, oligosaccharides (specific fibers) tend to be the component of wheat or soy that need to be avoided when following a low FODMAP diet. There are processing methods that reduce the oligosaccharides and make specific soy or wheat based foods suitable for the low FODMAP diet. Tofu and sourdough breads that are made authentically can make good examples of some low FODMAP foods.

Chapter Six: Natural Methods to Reduce Irritable Bowel Syndrome Symptoms

Drinking ample amounts of water

Experts always recommend your everyday intake of water should be of 2-3 liters, at the very least. And that is just for you to maintain a healthy digestive tract. But if you suffer from irritable bowel syndrome, then the intake of water is required to be of 3 liters at the very least, on a daily basis. As has been mentioned already, it is just as vital to know when your water intakes should happen. Bear in mind that you are not supposed to flood the digestive system with liquid or water intake right before or after taking your meals. This is so that it does not slow down or interfere with the digestion process in any manner.

Water ensures you are hydrated throughout the course of the day, and makes sure that your stools are properly loosened up. This way they do not put a lot of pressure on your bowel during their passing.

Peppermint oil based supplements

There are a lot of people who often find some solace by using peppermint oil. If peppermint oil supplements are taken twice in a day, they can be highly beneficial. Pace them between your meals as they are known to properly deal with or reduce problems like flatulence, along with reducing pains related Irritable Bowel Syndrome. Not only that, but peppermint tea has also been known as an enhancer of digestion that also relieves you from problems such as chronic constipation. But it is advisable that you consult your physician before you consume any peppermint oil based supplements as it could cause underlying conditions like acid reflux, which could make your condition even worse. It is best to consult your physician first.

Reduce your levels of stress

Stress is one of the major contributing factors in a lot of problems and disturbances that we face in our lives, be it mental or physical. It is important to have a stress free life in order to keep irritable bowel problems at bay. When the anxiety levels heighten due to everyday stress, it can end up aggravating any other problems that could be underlying.

When leading a stressful kind of life, you should consider engaging in activities such as meditation or yoga. These are activities through which you can maintain a state of mind that is both healthy and peaceful. Also, it would help to treat yourself to various herbal teas, spas, and other similar relaxing activities on a regular basis.

Try not to be sedentary

If you have been leading a lifestyle that is rather sedentary, then it is high time you literally moved your rear end. Try making some form of physical exercise or activity a part of your everyday routine. If you have a job or work life that requires you to sit in a single position or posture for prolonged periods of time – be careful! Do make sure that you get up at least once every hour, and also make sure you keep moving. Keep in mind that when you engage in any physical activity or exercise, it automatically makes your body relieve itself from stress and worries. In fact, it will also end up flooding you with positive and brighter feelings that will make you feel more energized. When you are actually happy and feeling energized in life, it makes your body cure itself a lot faster as opposed to the times you are not.

Consuming herbal teas to alleviate Irritable Bowel Syndrome symptoms

According to a lot of studies, herbal teas have been known to have soothing effects on your body as a whole and they also alleviate symptoms related to Irritable Bowel Syndrome. Teas especially like peppermint tea and chamomile teas have gained a lot of popularity with individuals who suffer from irritable bowel issues. There isn't much to it really; all it involves is pouring a glass of water into an appropriate pan and then bringing it to a boil. Next, add about a teaspoon of chamomile tea and let it steep for around 10-15 minutes before you drink it. Letting chamomile teas steep for that long ensures extracting maximum amounts of flavor of the tea and, at the same time, giving you a calming effect.

Chapter Seven: Meal Plan Ideas

Until you get to the part where some truly amazing recipes have been compiled for you, here's a typical framework of low FODMAP meal plan ideas. They are meant to give you a general idea about meals related to the diet. It will help you acquaint yourself to the structure, and later when you've gone through the recipes, you can adjust your meal plans as per your taste preferences. But it doesn't hurt to know how to structure a meal plan, so here's one to better your understanding of a low FODMAP diet meal plan –

Sunday

Breakfast – omelet with bell peppers, cheddar cheese, olives, tomatoes, and spinach, paired with some coffee and gluten-free toast that has been smeared with some spread that is lactose free.

Lunch – sandwich that has been assembled with turkey (no high fructose corn syrup), alfalfa sprouts, Swiss cheese, mayonnaise that is HCFS-free, and gluten free bread. A glass of lemonade, some sunflower seeds with corn chips to snack on.

Dinner – Roasted beef and potatoes baked with rosemary and salt, along with a salad made with tomatoes, lettuce and balsamic vinegar dressing that contains no HCFS, and a glass of peppermint tea – weak.

Monday

Breakfast – smoothie made with frozen strawberries, almond milk, flax seeds and banana, green tea.

Lunch – make a sandwich using gluten free bread, Swiss cheese, alfalfa sprouts, mayonnaise and leftover roast beef, gluten free crackers, a glass of lemonade and cantaloupe for snacking options.

Dinner – baked chicken that has been cooked in sunflower seed oil, pepper, salt, green part of spring onions, and topped with a sauce that is free of HFCS. Serve over brown rice and some steamed green beans along with almonds that have been sliced.

Tuesday

Breakfast – oatmeal with brown sugar and blueberries, coffee.

Lunch – Take some left over baked chicken and pair it with a salad made with tomatoes, spinach, an HFCS free raspberry vinaigrette, and mandarin oranges; for snacking purposes go for sunflower seeds, gluten free crackers, and a glass of limeade.

Dinner – a stir-fry made with pork, carrots, cabbage, bamboo shoots, green beans and water chestnuts served with brown rice; peppermint tea.

Wednesday

Breakfast – smoothie made from frozen blueberries, almond milk, chia seeds and banana; coffee.

Lunch – a salad assembled with tomatoes, tuna, slices of almonds, spinach, and HFCS free raspberry vinaigrette. For snacking go for – strawberries with some lactose free yogurt or a cup of black tea – weak.

Dinner – prepare a beef stew with foods and veggies allowed on the low FODMAP diet. Avoid using onions or tomato paste.

Thursday

Breakfast – oatmeal with almond milk, banana slices, and brown sugar; coffee.

Lunch – Sandwich assembled with gluten free bread, Swiss cheese, HFCS free mayonnaise, turkey and mustard. For snacking go for – cantaloupe and limeade.

Dinner – make some chicken adobo without any of the food ingredients that you are supposed to avoid. Salsa made with tomatoes, green onion, limes, parsley and greens; lemon tea.

Friday

Breakfast – smoothie made from frozen strawberries, banana, almond milk, and flax seeds; a cup of coffee.

Lunch – melted cheddar cheese on gluten free chips along with bell peppers, olives and diced tomatoes; and for snacking go for gluten free chips with some salsa; a glass of limeade.

Dinner – pan fry some shrimp in sunflower oil, top it with some lemon. Top that over brown rice and stir fry veggies like cabbage, carrots, bean sprouts and green beans.

Saturday

Breakfast – gluten free waffles topped with (no HFCS) maple syrup and blueberries; a cup of coffee.

Lunch – a salad assembled using bell peppers, alfalfa sprouts, lettuce, tomato, and a dressing that is HFCS free. For snacking opt for – strawberries with yogurt that is lactose free, a cup of black tea – weak.

Dinner – top some slices of baked ham with chunks of pineapple; bake potatoes using salt, rosemary leaves and sunflower seed oil; bake green beans and top them with slices of almonds.

Chapter Eight: The Low FODMAP Diet and Weight Loss

Losing weight can be a real struggle for a lot of people; more so if you are restricted by the limitations set by a low FODMAP diet. If you ever thought losing weight was not possible while on a low FODMAP diet, then read on, some tips have been compiled just for you –

Practice being lenient towards yourself

This is one of the most important tips that you could come across. All of us are humans and it is a human thing to make mistakes. Munched on a bar of chocolate you should not have? It happens. Consumed a slice of cake that is not low FODMAP although you have been trying real hard to stick to the diet? That happens as well. However, what you should really avoid doing when such scenarios occur is get mad or annoyed at yourself. You should also avoid talking down to yourself because, if that happens, it becomes incredibly easy to give up and let everything just go. Yes, it is much easier said than done. But it is easy to get frustrated when you are already under the wrath of IBS symptoms while battling it out with the help of a low FODMAP diet. So, relax! If you slip – pick up right where you left instead of giving up and letting all your efforts be for nothing.

Maintain a food diary for several days or a week

Maintaining a food diary has many benefits – it can give you some really valuable insights be it for your weight loss or for your IBS symptoms. In fact, there are many apps you could use for this purpose, but you could do it the pen and paper way as well! As mentioned in some earlier chapters, maintaining a diary to track your Irritable Bowel Syndrome can be really helpful and most importantly – insightful.

Not only can you jot down your Irritable Bowel Syndrome symptoms to figure out what triggers them but also to keep track of how much you are eating in a day. When you keep a track of these details, you can track how many extra calories you are consuming. From some chocolate consumed here, a cookie or two there, a slice of cheese somewhere, etc. You might be under the impression that being on a low FODMAP diet directly insinuates you are on a healthy diet – sure. But even the portion matters when you are eating healthy. Using any fitness-based apps to track your calories is a great way to gain some insight into how you might be gaining weight - also how and where you need to add some extra consideration to control these calories.
Instead of tracking the calories for every meal you eat, try tracking them for your calories and meals for around a week. When you start calculating your

calories for whatever and whenever you eat, it may end up as an unhealthy obsession.

Adding more fruits and veggies to your snacks and over all meals

How do you ensure you are consuming enough fruits and veggies? Well, you could start by adding a piece of low FODMAP fruit to your breakfast. Snack on another piece or two of fruit later. Always aim to add at least 150g to 200g of veggies to your dinner. If you use different types of vegetables, then getting to this amount will be fairly easy for you. You could opt for adding one or two types of veggies that contain no FODMAPs along with one type of veggie that is low in FODMAPs. What this will do is that it will help ensure you are not overloading on FODMAPs in any manner.

To give you an example – red bell pepper and tomato with ½ cup of zucchini that is limited. Other options are - lettuce with cucumber and tomato, with 1/8 of an avocado (also limited), pumpkin with a cup of broccoli heads (limited as well).
As for your lunch options, try adding about 100g to 150g of vegetables to your lunch. You could also consume them like snacks and you will easily be consuming 250g to 300g of veggies every day! You can put some tomato, lettuce, or cucumber in your sandwich as a lunch option. Or you could even snack on small tomatoes and slices of carrot, bell

pepper, or cucumber for a snack. Not only are veggies good for your overall health but they are also fulfilling and hardly contain any calories. So that is a win-win situation to consume a lot of them!

Focus on the can haves and not the can't haves of your diet

If you really do want to lose weight while consuming low FODMAP foods, then it becomes fairly simple and easy to focus on everything you do not want to eat. Or more importantly – cannot eat. However, focusing on the negatives of this diet is most definitely not going to ease things up for you. Instead, try focusing on everything you can consume. Go through the list of foods that you are allowed to have. Pore over the recipes in this book, look through all the meal options available to you, and you will realize not all is lost. In fact, a lot has been opened up to you. The low FODMAP way of eating might be a different and restrictive one - or you might think so - but wait until you go through all the recipes in this book. You will find out that the low FODMAP style of eating need not be as restrictive as you might perceive it to be. In fact, once you know your way around, you get to experiment a lot. Think not of the restrictions but of the possibilities! There are a lot of healthy recipes out there for you to try out in order to lose weight. Or – you could use the recipes in this book with a dash of cleverness and portion control, to let them fit into your weight loss regime.

Planning ahead

When and how does consuming a low FODMAP diet go wrong? When you do not plan ahead! And when you don't plan ahead what happens is that you end up snacking on something that is neither low FODMAP nor FODMAP diet related while on the go. Or you might even go for fries while deciding on dinner! This is why it is so important to make some time over the weekend, sit and plan a few things out for the week. When you are making your grocery lists, make sure you do not buy anything that is not a part of the low FODMAP diet. More importantly – it is not unhealthy even if it's on the low FODMAP list of foods you are allowed to eat.

Plan out what you want to cook this week. Try choosing meals that are quick, easy and healthy. If you are going to have a busy and hectic work schedule, then ensure there's always some low FODMAP meal in your freeze. You can always cook a bit extra when preparing rice or pasta dishes, then freeze it. Think of the times you don't have a lot of work or just want to relax for a bit. Instead of spending all your time in the kitchen, then you could just take out your low FODMAP frozen meal and heat it up. This way, you have a meal that is healthy, and even on days when you do not feel like cooking, you have something to rely on.

Chapter Nine: Tips for Eating out when on the Low FODMAP Diet

First of all – being on a low FODMAP diet should not mean you should limit or miss out of any kind of social activities. Eating can be difficult and tricky when you are following a low FODMAP diet, but it is, in fact, a very possible thing! In fact, being on this diet should not stop you from indulging in such activities. Being around friends and family, enjoying a nice meal – these are things almost everyone enjoys doing. That is why it is essential you do not miss out on any of these simple pleasures of life.

Here are some tips that will help you with eating out when you are on a low FODMAP diet –

It's the low FODMAP, not a no FODMAP diet!

The low FODMAP diet is all about placing a limit on the quantity of FODMAPs you consume, and not about excluding them from your diet entirely. In fact, it is not an absolute disaster if you end up consuming more FODMAPs every now and then. But it's important that to keep your Irritable Bowel Syndrome symptoms under control, you are not crossing any limitations in extreme manners. When you eat out, be prepared to experience a few more symptoms than you usually do. Try to limit the FODMAPs that you consume as much as possible. It may not be too dramatic if you end up having slightly more than your normal amount. As per a lot of IBS sufferers, they are fine with this because they claim it will only result in a bit of bloating and discomfort later.

There is one thing most people tend to forget. Even people who do not suffer from Irritable Bowel Syndrome tend to get bloated a bit when they consume things they normally do not eat or eat only when eating out. So, being a little bloated following a meal that was eaten out is not something that is going to get too dramatic.

However, what you really need to avoid it consuming large amounts of FODMAPs. That could result in being in pain for the days to come. There is a difference between a bit of bloating and upsetting your stomach entirely.

Ensure checking the menu beforehand

It can be really difficult for followers of the low FODMAP diet to select a restaurant right on the spot. That's why it is a lot smarter to check and go through the menus of restaurants before you end up going there so you can go to a restaurant based on their menu. It can be pretty upsetting if you are in a restaurant only to realize there isn't anything that you can eat. In fact, some types of restaurants like tapas or Italian tend to have either little or absolutely no low FODMAP options available. You really should avoid trying such restaurants.

This is why it is important you go over a restaurant's menu beforehand. Just find it online and pore over it for a minute; that one-minute is not going to cost you anything. However, eating at a place that does not have any low FODMAP friendly foods – could cost you a lot of pain for the next few days to come.

Informing a restaurant of your intolerances

When you have selected a restaurant, it is a smart move to inform them of your intolerances before you go there. There even are individuals who send lists of low FODMAP foods to a restaurant before visiting. If that restaurant is accepting and is willing enough to adapt some meals for you as per the list – bingo!

Not everyone is comfortable going through all of these things, but that is a choice that you are completely free to make. Instead of sending lists – there are also those who choose to inform the restaurant of all the things they react to. These could be anything you are aware you react to. They can be anything from garlic, onion, wheat and apple. Instead of saying wheat you could also say gluten since a lot of places are aware of how they should be dealing with gluten a lot better.

Pick the dishes that are the safes and try making adaptations if required

When you are in a restaurant and you have already informed them of your dietary intolerances, it is time for you to choose a dish. Next up, you can tell the restaurant that there are a lot more ingredients that are high FODMAP that you could avoid. Make sure you check for these ingredients as you are going through the menu. If at all possible – pick a dish that contains no ingredients that are high FODMAP. In case that is not possible – simply ask if they can substitute that ingredient with something or simply leave it out entirely. For example – dressings and sauces can often be quite problematic. If you are going to have a salad, simply ask them to replace the salad's dressing with a bit of olive oil. In this way, you can come up with a dish yourself that is low FODMAP.

Be watchful of the serving size, sugar, and fat

After being mindful about FODMAPs, you need to be very careful and watchful of not only your serving size but also the amounts of sugar and fat that you consume. Sugar and fat have been known as triggers of Irritable Bowel Syndrome. Too much of either could cause a lot of problems so it is better to avoid both.

You've upset your stomach – what now?

It is a highly probable scenario for things to go wrong when you eat out but later end up in a lot of pain. It can be quite upsetting, but yes it can happen occasionally. What you can do when this occurs is to go back to the basics. Over the next few days, try choosing meals you tolerate well. This way you can try calming down your stomach again.

Chapter Ten: Reincorporating FODMAPs Back into Your Dietary Habits

The low FODMAP diet is not a diet that is supposed to be followed for a lifetime – isn't that amazing? But yes – it is a diet that has been designed in order to identify the causes behind symptoms related to Irritable Bowel Syndrome. It will help you gain knowledge regarding how you can craft your diet in the future. Or alter it to suit and manage your condition a lot better than before once you are done with the low FODMAP diet

So, once you have been on the FODMAP diet for 6 to 8 weeks – what next? To continue with it or go back to the regular diet you used to be on?

Okay, so, first of all – how are you feeling? Are you feeling better? If even after being on the low FODMAP diet, you do not feel any better, and then it is best to re-evaluate your food intake. See if there have been any accidental slip-ups at any point. What triggers your symptoms may be different from what triggers another person's irritable bowel syndrome symptoms. There are those whose bodies are unable to tolerate citrusy fruits. But most of the citrus fruits are on the "can be eaten" section of FODMAP food lists. There are even things to consider like – gluten. Since the low FODMAP diet is not gluten free, it is possible that gluten could be the root cause of your symptoms.

Do you consume meals that are bigger? Even this could be an issue since the low FODMAP diet specifically encourages the intake of smaller meals. It also advises consuming meals in smaller quantities albeit more frequently throughout the course of the day.

In fact, it could also be something as simple as vitamins, medicine, lipstick and gum. Or even the lip-gloss that you use could be the reason that is causing your bowel related problems. Keep a check on anything and everything that goes near the mouth, even a partner whom you kiss.

After being on a FODMAP free diet, if you are beginning to feel better, then you might feel courageous enough to start testing out FODMAPs in your diet. Then here are some of the next steps you would need to take –

> 1. Make sure you carefully select a FODMAP group that you are interested in testing out to reintroduce into your diet. Try choosing the one that you miss more than the rest. A lot of people will start off by reintroducing fructans, due to the spices and wheat, whereas someone else would

not choose that since they figured out and grew accustomed to substituting and making clever replacements. When it comes to spices, onion and garlic, for example, using asafetida powder. There is also gluten – for some, after going gluten free for several years, they end up no longer cravings foods like baked goods, etc. contrary to some who would be full of gluten related cravings. Then there are those who would be dying for some lactose based foods.

2. So once you have selected a FODMAP group that you have decided to reintroduce in your diet, it is time to choose how you want to try or attempt it. Try picking a food you have missed, take it in a small quantity when you are having dinner. If you are wondering why dinner specifically – that is because there is a chance that it might not be successful. Then you will most probably end up sleeping through most of the probable symptoms and that won't end up ruining your day. If you want to choose lactose as the group to reintroduce, then having a 10-12 oz glass

of milk in the morning during breakfast would not be a good idea since it would be a large quantity and you might even end up feeling really sick by the time it's lunchtime. Instead, try having a small portion of some lactose based food during dinner. As mentioned earlier, it would be a lot more convenient to sleep through the symptoms than to let them affect your entire day which, let's face it – would be very discouraging if you are just beginning to gather your guts (no pun intended!) to attempt reintroducing FODMAPS into your diet.

3. Once you have courageously consumed the FODMAP group, try observing all your symptoms as closely as you can. Make sure you make a record of all of these details related to the symptoms. Maintain a diary of everything you have attempted. Write down when exactly you have attempted them, and mention all the symptoms in details that you have encountered, if any. Keep a track of these for the next 24 hours. Tracking your symptoms is very important.

4. If you are not successful in your tries and some or all of your Irritable Bowel Syndrome symptoms start making a comeback, then hey! You have most certainly discovered one of the triggers associated with your IBS, including the quantity. This in itself is a great achievement. If it possible, test an even smaller amount of the FODMAP food later that day. Then make notes of all your symptoms once you start feeling better and the symptoms have subsided.

5. In case you are successful in the first reintroduction that you attempted, try something pretty similar in quantity. Make sure that belongs to that very FODMAP group. Once again, try it the very next day, and then start tracking your symptoms once again. If this ends up being unsuccessful then refer to the point preceding this one – point no. 4.

6. If your second test ends up being successful – then great! It means you can consume the food you tried during dinner fairly safely. Now what you need to do is try having that food item slightly earlier, say around lunch. Then carefully track your symptoms in a detailed manner once again. If this attempt ends up falling through, then refer to point no. 4. It is pretty common to be fine with the same quantity and amount of foods during dinnertime but not when it comes to lunch. This has been the case for quite a few individuals. They had no symptoms when consuming their gluten free mac and cheese in small portions at dinner, but ended up getting stomach pains and also bloating around 4-5 after they attempted consuming it for lunch. This, however, was not noticed when they tried testing it at dinnertime, as they slept and the next morning – and felt just fine.

7. Succeeded once again? Great! So, every time your attempt is successful and you do not feel any kind of symptoms, you know what to do. You repeat with adding

additional amounts of that specific FODMAP group's food to your intake of meals. Gradually, you will reach point where you will observe that this specific FODMAP group does not affect you. Or you might be able to figure out the limit or portions you can safely consume.

8. Once you have successfully figured out the quantity of that specific FODMAP group's food that you can consume safely – congratulations! You can proceed to test out the next one that you prefer. After around 3 months you will be aware of what and how much of it you can tolerate. This will help you build your diet for you to use in the future.

Bear in mind that the low FODMAP diet (and any other method of treatment) is not going to 'cure' your Irritable Bowel Syndrome as some people might claim. Sadly, so far, there is no way to cure Irritable Bowel Syndrome. In fact, in order to find that, they would first need to figure out the cause behind it, which has not been done so far. The low FODMAP diet's goal is to help you manage

Irritable Bowel Syndrome's symptoms through your everyday diet. This has worked for a lot of people really well.

Chapter Eleven: Breakfast Recipes

Baked Oatmeal Cups

Serves: 6
Ingredients:
- 1 egg
- ¼ cup water
- 1 teaspoon vanilla extract
- 1 ¼ cups old fashioned oats
- ½ teaspoon ground cinnamon
- 1 tablespoon vegetable oil like canola or grape seed oil
- ½ cup lactose free milk
- 2 ½ tablespoons brown sugar
- 1 teaspoon baking powder

Optional toppings: Use any
- Strawberries, sliced
- Mini semi-sweet chocolate chips
- Almonds or walnuts, chopped
- Cranberries

Method:
1. Place paper liners in a 6-count muffin tin.
2. Add oil, eggs, milk and water into a bowl and whisk well.
3. Add rest of the ingredients and whisk well. Let it rest for 2-3 minutes. Mix again.

4. Divide the batter among the muffin cups. Place the toppings if using.
5. Bake in a preheated oven at 350 °F for 20-25 minutes. It should turn slightly brown on the edges when done.
6. Cool for a while and serve.

Breakfast Cereal Bars

Serves:

Ingredients:
- 2 tablespoons olive oil or coconut oil or butter
- ½ cup natural peanut butter
- 4 cups mini marshmallows without high fructose corn syrup
- 6 cups Mesa Sunrise cereal

Method:
1. Add the fat you are using and marshmallows into a large saucepan. Place saucepan over low heat.
2. Stir constantly until the marshmallows melt.
3. Stir in peanut butter. Stir constantly until smooth. Turn off the heat.
4. Stir in the cereal. Transfer the mixture into a square or rectangular pan. Place a parchment paper on top of the mixture and spread the mixture evenly into the pan, pressing lightly.
5. Refrigerate for 45-60 minutes.
6. Cut into bars and serve.

Breakfast Potatoes

Serves: 4-6

Ingredients:
- 4 large Idaho potatoes, rinsed well
- ½ cup lactose free yogurt
- 4 tablespoons butter, softened
- 2/3 cup sharp cheddar cheese, grated
- 8 bacon strips
- 5-6 slices thin prosciutto
- Salt to taste
- Pepper to taste
- Baby arugula or spinach to top (optional)

Method:
1. Prick the outer surface of the potatoes with a fork at different places.
2. Bake in a preheated oven at 350 °F for 60-75 minutes or until tender.
3. Place the potatoes on your cutting board. Using a kitchen towel, hold the potatoes and cut each into 2 halves. Scoop the flesh of the potatoes and add into a bowl. Place the potatoes on a baking sheet.
4. Add butter, yogurt and cheese into the bowl of scooped potatoes and mash it until creamy. Fill this mixture into the potato cases.
5. Cook the eggs, bacon and prosciutto in a pan. Top over the potatoes.

6. Bake for 10minutes.
7. Serve hot garnished with baby arugula.

Blueberry Kiwi Minty Groovy Smoothie

Serves: 2

Ingredients:
- 1 cup frozen blueberries
- 2/3 cup lactose free yogurt
- A handful fresh mint leaves (12-15 leaves)
- 2 kiwifruits, peeled, chopped
- 2/3 cup water

Method:
1. Add all the ingredients into a blender and blend until smooth.
2. Pour into tall glasses and serve.

Pineapple Ginger Kale Smoothie

Serves: 2

Ingredients:
- 2 cups nondairy milk of your choice
- 1 ½ cups fresh or frozen pineapple chunks
- 2 inches fresh ginger, peeled, grated or ½ teaspoon dried ginger
- 1 orange, peeled, separated into segments, deseeded
- 2 cups kale
- 2 cups ice

Method:
1. Add all the ingredients into a blender and blend until smooth.
2. Pour into tall glasses and serve.

Potato Scones

Serves: 8

Ingredients:
- 1 ¾ pounds floury potatoes, peeled cubed
- ½ teaspoon salt
- 1 cup self-raising gluten free flour + extra for dusting
- Butter or oil to grease

Method:
1. Place a pot half filled with water over high heat.
2. When it begins to boil, add potatoes and cook until tender.
3. Drain and add potatoes into a bowl. Mash with a potato masher until smooth.
4. Add flour and salt and mix to form dough.
5. Divide the mixture into 6 equal portions.
6. Dust your countertop with some flour. Using a rolling pin, roll into rounds of about ½ cm thick. Cut each into 4 wedges.
7. Place a skillet over medium heat. Add oil or butter. When pan heats, place 3-4 pieces of scones and cook for 3-4 minutes. Flip sides and cook the other side too.
8. Repeat the above step and cook the remaining in batches.
9. Serve with scrambled eggs.

Chapter Twelve: Snack Recipes

Carrot and Parsnip Chips

Serves:
Ingredients:
- 2 large or medium carrots, peeled, trimmed
- 2 large or 4 medium parsnips, peeled, trimmed
- Olive oil cooking spray
- 2 teaspoons thyme leaves, chopped (optional)
- Salt to taste

Method:
1. Make long strips of the carrots and parsnips using a 'Y' shaped vegetable peeler.
2. Spread it on a greased baking sheet. Spray with cooking spray.
3. Sprinkle salt and thyme leaves.
4. Bake in a preheated oven at 325 °F for 35 minutes. Turn the chips a couple of times while baking.

Bacon Wrapped Pineapple

Serves: 10

Ingredients:
- 5 slices precooked bacon, halved
- ½ tablespoon pure maple syrup
- 10 bite size pieces pineapple

Method:
1. Place bacon slices in the microwave and microwave on high for 15 seconds.
2. Place bacon slices on a baking sheet. Place a piece of pineapple on each slice of bacon at one end. Wrap and fasten with a toothpick. Drizzle maple syrup over it.
3. Bake in a preheated oven at 350 °F for 5-10 minutes.

Roasted Chickpeas
Serves: 8 (¼ cup each)

Ingredients:
- 2 cans chickpeas, drained, rinsed
- ½ teaspoon freshly ground pepper
- ½ teaspoon salt
- 1 teaspoon dried rosemary, crushed
- ½ teaspoon smoked sweet paprika
- 2 teaspoons olive oil
- 1 teaspoon garlic powder
- ½ teaspoon dried thyme

Method:
1. Dry the chickpeas with a clean kitchen towel.
2. Add chickpeas into a bowl. Drizzle oil over it and toss well.
3. Sprinkle seasonings on top and toss until well coated.
4. Line a baking sheet with aluminum foil. Spread the chickpeas on it in a single layer.
5. Bake in a preheated oven at 450° F for about 30-45 minutes. Toss 2-3 times while it is baking. Bake until it is turning light brown in color.
6. Remove the baking sheet from the oven after 15-20 minutes.
7. Cool completely. Transfer into an airtight container and store until use.

Cucumber and Dill-infused Cottage Cheese Appetizer

Serves:

Ingredients:
- 2 large cucumbers, trimmed, cut into 1 ½ inch thick round slices
- 4 teaspoons garlic infused oil
- 2 scallions, thinly slice the green parts only, to garnish
- 1 ½ cups lactose free cottage cheese
- 4 teaspoons fresh dill, chopped or 1 teaspoon dried dill
- Coarsely ground pepper to taste

Method:
1. Place the cucumber rounds on a serving platter. Carefully scoop out some of the seeds and flesh from the cucumber rounds, keeping the base intact.
2. Mix together in a bowl, cottage cheese, dill and garlic infused oil. Divide the mixture and fill in the cucumber cases.
3. Sprinkle scallions and pepper powder and serve.

Chapter Thirteen: Lunch Recipes

Potato Salad with Anchovy and Quail's Eggs

Serves: 2
Ingredients:
- 8 quail's eggs
- 7 ounces new potatoes, halved or quartered, depending on the size
- 7 ounces green beans
- A handful fresh parsley, chopped
- Juice of a lemon
- 2 anchovies, finely chopped
- 2 tablespoons chopped chives

Method:
1. Place a pot over medium heat. Pour enough water to fill up to about ¾.
2. When it begins to boil, gently lower the eggs into the water. Let it simmer for 2 minutes and 15 seconds for soft boiled.
3. Remove the eggs with a slotted spoon and plunge in a bowl of cold water.
4. Add beans into the simmering water in the pot and cook for 4 minutes. Remove beans and submerge in a bowl of cold water.
5. Now add potatoes to the simmering water. Cook until tender. Discard the water and place potatoes in a colander. Let it cool.

6. Peel and halve the eggs.
7. Add potatoes, beans, anchovies, lemon juice, parsley and chives into a bowl and toss well.
8. Divide into individual plates. Place eggs on top and serve.

Low FODMAP Chicken Noodle Soup

Serves: 6-8

Ingredients:
- 4-6 cups low FODMAP chicken broth
- 2 cups chopped, cooked chicken breast
- Salt to taste
- Pepper to taste
- 4-6 cups water
- 4-8 ounces raw gluten free pasta / noodles like brown rice pasta fusilli

Method:
1. Pour broth and water into a pot. Place the pot over medium heat. Stir frequently.
2. When it begins to boil, add pasta, salt, pepper and chicken and cook until pasta is al dente.
3. Ladle into soup bowls and serve.

Egg Wraps

Serves: 2

Ingredients:
- 4 egg whites
- 2 eggs
- Pepper to taste
- Salt to taste
- Toppings of your choice that are low FODMAP friendly

Method:
1. Whisk together in a bowl, whites, eggs, salt and pepper.
2. Place a nonstick pan over medium heat. Spray with cooking spray. Pour half the egg mixture.
3. Cook for 2-3 minutes. Flip sides and cook the other side too.
4. Carefully slide on to a plate. Place toppings of your choice and wrap. Serve right away.
5. Repeat the above 3 steps to make the other wrap.

Poached Egg Sandwich with Smoked Salmon

Serves: 2

Ingredients:
- 4 fresh eggs
- ¼ avocado
- Lemon juice to taste
- Rocket lettuce (optional)
- 3.5 ounces smoked salmon
- Pepper to taste
- Salt to taste
- 4 slices sourdough spelt bread

Method:
1. Add avocado, lemon juice, salt and pepper into a bowl and mash well with a fork.
2. Smear this on one side of the bread slices.
3. Place salmon on each of the slices. Place rocket leaves on top.
4. Place a pan of water over high heat. When the water begins to boil, lower heat. Crack the eggs in it and poach the eggs. Remove carefully and place over the sandwiches. Season with salt and pepper and serve.

Buckwheat Pancakes

Makes: 5-6

Ingredients:
- 3.5 ounces buckwheat flour
- A small pinch salt
- 10 ounces lactose free milk
- 1 egg, at room temperature
- Cooking spray
- Toppings of your choice that are low FODMOP friendly

Method:
1. Add buckwheat flour and salt into a bowl. Add egg and whisk until well combined.
2. Add milk, a little at a time and whisk well.
3. Place a nonstick pan or griddle over medium heat. Spray with cooking spray,
4. Pour about ¼ cup batter over it. Swirl the pan so that the batter spreads. Cook until the underside is golden brown. Flip sides and cook the other side too.
5. Place toppings of your choice and serve.

Chapter Fourteen: Dinner Recipes

Sweet and Sour Chicken

Serves: 8
Ingredients:
- 2 pounds chicken breasts, skinless, boneless, cut into 1 inch pieces
- 2 large eggs, beaten
- 1 cup coconut sugar or regular white sugar
- 4 tablespoons coconut aminos or tamari
- ½ cup chicken stock
- 2 cups pineapple chunks
- 1 cup arrowroot starch or cornstarch
- ½ cup coconut oil
- ½ cup apple cider vinegar or white wine or rice vinegar
- ½ cup ketchup or Low FODMAP ketchup
- 2 red peppers, cut into 1 inch squares
- 6 spring onions, green parts only, thinly sliced
- Oil, as required

Method:
1. To make sauce: Add coconut sugar, coconut aminos, vinegar, stock and ketchup into a saucepan. Place the saucepan over medium heat. Stir frequently.
2. When it begins to boil, lower heat and let it simmer.

3. Add chicken into the bowl of eggs. Stir until well coated. Sprinkle some arrowroot over it. Toss and sprinkle again. Toss until the pieces are well coated.
4. Place a large skillet over medium heat. Add oil. When the oil is heated, add chicken and cook until slightly crisp on all the sides.
5. Add red pepper and pineapple and stir. Cook until chicken is brown and tender from inside.
6. Pour the simmering sauce over the chicken. Stir and lower heat.
7. Cover and simmer for 3-5 minutes. Turn off heat.
8. Add green onions and stir. Serve with rice.

Baked Lemon Pepper Chicken & Rice

Serves: 6

Ingredients:
- 6 chicken breasts, skinless, boneless, thinly sliced
- 6 tablespoons butter or vegan butter, melted
- 1 ½ cups basmati rice
- 2 tablespoons lemon pepper seasoning or to taste
- 28 ounces chicken broth
- 1 teaspoon salt (do not add if the chicken broth is salted)

Method:
1. Sprinkle lemon pepper seasoning all over the chicken.
2. Add butter into a large baking dish. Swirl the dish so that butter spreads all over.
3. Place chicken in the dish. Cover the dish with foil.
4. Bake in a preheated oven at 350° F for about 30-45 minutes or until tender. Flip sides after about 15-18 minutes during baking.
5. Remove chicken from the dish and place on a plate. Cover the plate and keep it warm.
6. Add broth, rice and salt into the same dish. Cover the dish with foil.

7. Bake for 30 minutes or until rice is cooked. Place chicken on top. Cover with foil.
8. Bake for another 15-20 minutes.
9. Serve hot.

Beef Skillet Supper

Serves: 6

Ingredients:
- 2 pounds grass fed ground beef
- 1 medium cabbage, sliced (optional)
- 2 teaspoons fresh ginger, peeled, grated
- 2 medium zucchinis, very thinly sliced, preferably with a mandolin slicer
- 2 scallions, green parts only, thinly sliced, to garnish
- 3 cups white sweet potato, diced
- 2 large carrots, very thinly sliced, preferably with a mandolin slicer
- A handful fresh cilantro or parsley, chopped to garnish
- 2 teaspoons duck fat or bacon fat or lard or more if required
- 6 tablespoons coconut aminos
- Sea salt to taste

Method:
1. Place a large skillet over medium high heat (preferably cast iron skillet). Add fat.
2. When fat melts, add beef and cook until light brown.
3. Stir in coconut aminos, ginger, sweet potato and cabbage.

4. Cover and cook until sweet potatoes are tender. Stir occasionally. Remove from heat.
5. Add carrots and zucchini and stir until well combined. Cover and let it sit for a few minutes.
6. Place the skillet back on heat for a couple of minutes if you like the carrots and zucchini more cooked.
7. Divide into plates. Sprinkle scallion, cilantro and salt and serve.

Sardine Spaghetti with Tomato- Caper Sauce

Serves: 6

Ingredients:
- 4 tablespoons extra- virgin olive oil or garlic infused oil, divided
- 4 cans (4.35 ounces each) sardines, drained, de-boned if required
- 1/3 cup gluten free breadcrumbs
- 6 ounces spinach leaves
- ½ teaspoon red chili flakes or to taste
- 2 tablespoons drained capers, roughly chopped
- ½ - 1 avocado, peeled, pitted, chopped
- Freshly ground pepper to taste
- Salt to taste
- 5-6 scallions, green parts only, thinly sliced
- 2 cans (14.5 ounces each) petite or regular diced tomatoes
- 12 ounces gluten free spaghetti
- Lemon wedges to serve

Method:
1. Place a large skillet over medium heat. Add 4 teaspoons oil. When the oil is heated, add breadcrumbs and sauté until it is toasted lightly. Stir frequently.

2. Sprinkle salt and pepper and stir. Remove the breadcrumbs from the skillet and place in a bowl
3. Place the skillet back over heat. Add 2 teaspoons oil. When the oil is heated, add spinach and pepper and sauté until it wilts. Stir frequently. Remove the spinach and place in another bowl.
4. Place the skillet back over heat. Add 2 tablespoons oil. When the oil is heated, add scallions and chili flakes and sauté until it wilts.
5. Stir in the tomatoes with its juices. Increase the heat to medium high and let it cook until slightly thick. Stir occasionally.
6. Add capers and stir. Turn off the heat.
7. Cook spaghetti until al dente, following the directions on the package. Drain and add the pasta back into the cooked pot.
8. Set aside ½ cup of the cooked sauce (it can be used in some other recipe) and add rest of the sauce into the pot. Also add sardines and spinach and mix gently until well combined. Place over medium heat for a couple of minutes until hot.

9. Serve with breadcrumbs sprinkled on top. Also top with avocado and lemon wedges and serve.

Spiced Quinoa with Almonds and Feta

Serves: 6

Ingredients:
- 1 ½ tablespoons olive oil
- ¾ teaspoon turmeric
- 2.6 ounces flaked toasted almonds
- ½ cup parsley, chopped
- 2 tablespoons lemon juice or to taste
- 1 ½ teaspoons ground coriander
- 16 ounces quinoa, rinsed
- 5.3 ounces feta cheese, crumbled
- 4 cups boiling water

Method:
1. Place a large skillet over medium heat. Add oil. When the oil is heated, add turmeric and coriander powders and sauté for a few seconds until aromatic.
2. Add quinoa and stir-fry for a minute or so. You will be able to hear mild sounds of the quinoa popping.
3. Pour water and stir. Lower heat and cook until all the water has been absorbed and quinoa is tender.

4. Cool for a few minutes. Add rest of the ingredients and fluff gently and mix into it.
5. Serve either warm or cold.

Vegan Coconut Green Curry

Serves: 3

Ingredients:
- 1 teaspoon coconut oil or garlic infused oil
- 1 medium potato, peeled, cut into 1 inch cubes
- 1 cup spinach, shredded
- 1 small head broccoli, cut into florets
- 1 small courgette, chopped
- ½ inch ginger, peeled, minced
- ½ cup coconut milk
- ½ teaspoon ground cumin
- ¼ teaspoon red chili flakes
- ½ teaspoon ground turmeric
- 1 teaspoon lime juice
- A handful fresh cilantro, chopped (optional)
- A fistful cashews, chopped (optional)
- ½ cup water
- Salt to taste

Method:
1. Place a skillet over medium heat. Add oil. When the oil is heated, add ginger, turmeric and cumin and sauté for a few seconds until fragrant.
2. Add potatoes and sauté for a while. Sprinkle some water if the potatoes are getting stuck to the bottom of the pan.

3. Add broccoli and courgette and stir. Stir in coconut milk, salt and water.
4. Cover and cook until the vegetables are soft. Turn off the heat.
5. Add spinach, lime juice and chili flakes. Stir and cover for a few minutes.
6. Taste and adjust the lime, salt and chili flakes if necessary.
7. Sprinkle cilantro and cashew on top and serve.

Spicy Potato Pie

Serves: 6-8

Ingredients:
- 6 large potatoes, peeled, grated
- 1-2 red chilies, finely chopped
- 1 ½ tablespoons cooking oil
- 9 rashers bacon
- 6 eggs
- Salt to taste
- Pepper to taste
- 5 spring onions, green parts only, thinly sliced
- 3 teaspoons garlic infused oil
- 1 ½ red bell peppers, finely chopped
- 1 ½ bags baby spinach leaves, cut into thin strips
- ¼ cup rice flour
- ¼ cup tapioca flour, mixed

Method:
1. Place a skillet over medium heat. Add cooking oil and garlic infused oil. When the oils are heated, add chili and spring onions and sauté until tender.
2. Add bacon and cook for a while. Turn off heat. When cool enough to handle chop bacon into chunks.

3. Squeeze the potatoes of excess moisture. Add into a bowl. Add rest of the ingredients and mix well.
4. Transfer into a greased tart pan. Spread it evenly.
5. Bake in a preheated oven at 350° F for about 30-45 minutes.

Chapter Fifteen: Dessert Recipes

Banana Ice Cream

Serves: 10-12

Ingredients:
- 2 cans (14 ounces each) light coconut milk
- 2 teaspoons vanilla bean paste or extract
- 4 bananas, peeled, sliced
- ½ cup dark chocolate chips (optional)

Method:
1. Pour 1½ cans of coconut milk into ice an ice cube tray. Freeze until firm. Chill the remaining coconut milk.
2. Place bananas on a freezer safe tray and freeze until firm.
3. Add frozen bananas, coconut milk ice cubes, vanilla and coconut milk into a blender. Pulse until creamy.
4. Scoop into bowls. Sprinkle chocolate chips on top and serve.

Chocolate Peanut Butter Chia Pudding

Serves: 6-8 (1/3 cup each)

Ingredients:
- ½ cup chia seeds
- 2 tablespoons natural creamy peanut butter
- 2 tablespoons pure maple syrup
- 2 tablespoons cocoa powder, unsweetened
- 2 cups canned light coconut milk

Method:
1. Add all the ingredients into a jar with a lid or use a mason's jar.
2. Close the lid and shake the jar vigorously.
3. Uncover and stir with a spoon. Cover and shake the jar vigorously once more.
4. Chill for 4-6 hours.
5. Serve as it is or serve with fruits.

Frosted Biscotti

Serves:

Ingredients:
- 3 tablespoons butter, at room temperature
- 2 eggs
- 3 teaspoons baking powder
- 3 teaspoons vegetable oil
- 2 teaspoons almond extract
- 2 teaspoons vanilla extract
- 1 cup sugar
- 3 cups gluten free all-purpose flour blend
- 2/3 cup lactose free milk

For icing:
- 1 ½ -2 cups confectioner's sugar
- 1 teaspoon vanilla extract
- 4 tablespoons butter, at room temperature
- 2-3 teaspoons lactose free milk

Method:
1. Add butter and sugar into a mixing bowl. Beat with an electric mixer until smooth and creamy.
2. Add eggs, one at a time and beat well each time.
3. Mix together flour and baking powder and add into the bowl. Mix until well combined.
4. Add oil, vanilla and almond extracts and mix well.

5. Line a large baking sheet with parchment paper. You 2 baking sheets if required.
6. Drop large spoonful of batter on the prepared baking sheet. Leave a gap between 2 cookies.
7. Bake in a preheated oven at 350° F for about 20 minutes or until the edges are light brown.
8. Remove from the oven and let it cool for 5-8 minutes on the baking sheet. Loosen the cookies with a metal spatula. Cool completely.
9. Meanwhile, make the icing as follows: Add 1 cup confectioner's sugar, vanilla, butter and milk into a bowl and whisk well. Add remaining sugar and beat until creamy.
10. Spread a thin layer of the icing over the biscotti. Cut if desired and serve.
11. Store in an airtight container.

Chocolate Coconut Cookies

Serves:

Ingredients:
- 2 sticks butter, at room temperature
- 2 eggs
- 1 cup 60% cacao chocolate chips, melted, slightly cooled
- 1 cup whole grain brown rice flour
- ½ cup chopped, shredded sweetened coconut
- 2/3 cup granulated sugar
- 2 teaspoons vanilla extract
- 2 cups gluten free flour blend
- 2 teaspoons baking soda

Method:
1. Add butter and sugar into a mixing bowl. Beat with an electric mixer until smooth and creamy.
2. Add eggs, one at a time and beat well each time. Add chocolate and fold gently.
3. Mix together flour and baking powder and add into the bowl. Mix until well combined.
4. Add vanilla and mix well. Add coconut and mix to form dough.
5. Line a large baking sheet with parchment paper. You 2 baking sheets if required. Set aside.

6. Roll the dough into a cylindrical shape of about 2-½ inches diameter.
7. Wrap the dough with parchment paper and chill for 2-3 hours or until hard.
8. Remove the dough and place on your cutting board. Cut into 1/3 inch thick slices.
9. Place on the prepared baking sheet.
10. Bake in a preheated oven at 350° F for about 20 minutes or until the edges are light brown.
11. Remove from the oven and let it cool for 5-8 minutes on the baking sheet. Loosen the cookies with a metal spatula. Cool completely.
12. Store in an airtight container.

Chapter Sixteen: Dip Recipes

Arugula Feta Dip

Each serving is of ¼ cup
Ingredients:
- 8 cups baby arugula
- 4 tablespoons fresh lemon juice
- 28 ounces feta cheese
- 2-4 tablespoons garlic infused olive oil

Method:
1. Add all the ingredients into a blender and blend until smooth.
2. Transfer into a bowl and serve.

FODMAP Friendly Hummus

Each serving is of ¼ cup

Ingredients:
- 2 cans (14.5 ounces each) chickpeas, drained, rinsed
- 2 teaspoons ground cumin
- Water, as required
- 4 tablespoons lime juice
- 2 tablespoons garlic infused olive oil

Method:
1. Add all the ingredients into a blender and blend until smooth.
2. Transfer into a bowl and serve.

Berry Chia Jam

Makes: 2/3 cup

Ingredients:
- ½ cup strawberries, chopped
- 2 cups frozen wild blueberries
- 2 tablespoons chia seeds
- 3 tablespoons maple syrup
- 1 teaspoon vanilla extract

Method:
1. Add berries and maple syrup into a pan. Place the pan over medium heat.
2. In a while, the berries will begin to release its juices. Mash the berries with a potato masher.
3. Simmer until slightly thick. Add chia seeds and cook for a couple of minutes.
4. Turn off the heat. Let it cool for a while.
5. Transfer into a glass jar. Fasten the lid. Refrigerate until use.
6. It can store for 1 week in the refrigerator.

Conclusion

Once again, thank you for purchasing this book and making it to the very end of it! I trust it has proven to be to your benefit and you are all geared up to begin your journey with the low FODMAP diet.

Now that you know what Irritable Bowel Syndrome does to not only you but others as well and how to go about planning meals, eating out, the pitfalls to avoid, and all the easy and amazing low FODMAP recipes you can try out – there should be nothing to stop you from doing something about all the IBS symptoms you are suffering from.

Be careful about your meal intake, the portions, and whether the foods are on the FODMAP list or not. Start out basic; first acquaint yourself with all the IBS and low FODMAP diet related knowledge you have just acquired. I wish you luck!

Thank you.

Made in the USA
Middletown, DE
11 July 2019